| Name | |
|---|---|
| Address | |
| Phone No. | |
| Mobile No. | |
| Email | |
| Emergency Information | |
| Notes | |

## MEDICAL CONTACTS

| | |
|---|---|
| Name | |
| Type | |
| Hospital / Clinic | |
| Phone No. | |
| Mobile No. | |
| Email | |
| Notes | |

| | |
|---|---|
| Name | |
| Type | |
| Hospital / Clinic | |
| Phone No. | |
| Mobile No. | |
| Email | |
| Notes | |

| | |
|---|---|
| Name | |
| Type | |
| Hospital / Clinic | |
| Phone No. | |
| Mobile No. | |
| Email | |
| Notes | |

# SUPPORT GROUP

| Name | |
|---|---|
| Relationship | |
| Address | |
| Phone No. | |
| Mobile No. | |
| Email | |
| Notes | |

| Name | |
|---|---|
| Relationship | |
| Address | |
| Phone No. | |
| Mobile No. | |
| Email | |
| Notes | |

| Name | |
|---|---|
| Relationship | |
| Address | |
| Phone No. | |
| Mobile No. | |
| Email | |
| Notes | |

# SUPPORT GROUP

| | |
|---|---|
| Name | |
| Relationship | |
| Address | |
| Phone No. | |
| Mobile No. | |
| Email | |
| Notes | |

| | |
|---|---|
| Name | |
| Relationship | |
| Address | |
| Phone No. | |
| Mobile No. | |
| Email | |
| Notes | |

| | |
|---|---|
| Name | |
| Relationship | |
| Address | |
| Phone No. | |
| Mobile No. | |
| Email | |
| Notes | |

## MEDICAL HISTORY

| | |
|---|---|
| Date Of Birth | |
| Blood Type | |
| Chronic Conditions | |
| Food Allergies | |
| Medical Allergies | |
| Maintenance Medication | |
| Physician | |
| Notes | |

### Immunizations

| Date | Vaccinations | Hospital/Clinic | Notes |
|---|---|---|---|
| | | | |
| | | | |
| | | | |
| | | | |
| | | | |
| | | | |
| | | | |
| | | | |

Summary Of        Number Of Days

| Symptom / Illness/ Trigger | 1 | 2 | 3 | 4 | 5 | 6 | 7 | 8 | 9 | 10 |
|---|---|---|---|---|---|---|---|---|---|---|
| | | | | | | | | | | |
| | | | | | | | | | | |
| | | | | | | | | | | |
| | | | | | | | | | | |
| | | | | | | | | | | |
| | | | | | | | | | | |
| | | | | | | | | | | |
| | | | | | | | | | | |
| | | | | | | | | | | |
| | | | | | | | | | | |
| | | | | | | | | | | |

Summary Of        Number Of Days

| Symptom / Illness / Trigger | 1 | 2 | 3 | 4 | 5 | 6 | 7 | 8 | 9 | 10 |
|---|---|---|---|---|---|---|---|---|---|---|
| | | | | | | | | | | |
| | | | | | | | | | | |
| | | | | | | | | | | |
| | | | | | | | | | | |
| | | | | | | | | | | |
| | | | | | | | | | | |
| | | | | | | | | | | |
| | | | | | | | | | | |
| | | | | | | | | | | |
| | | | | | | | | | | |
| | | | | | | | | | | |

What does recovery mean to you?

## What does recovery mean to you?

**Stay Active**  **Date:**

Activity / Workout / Creativity / Hobbies
_____

_____
_____
_____
_____
_____
_____
_____

What are your goals ? (Work, Family & others)
_____

_____
_____
_____
_____
_____
_____

Steps towards your goals
_____

_____
_____
_____
_____
_____
_____
_____

**Date:**

## Triggers / Environment

## Symptoms

## Medication / Support System

**Stay Active**  **Date:**

## Activity / Workout / Creativity / Hobbies

_____
_____
_____
_____
_____
_____
_____

## What are your goals ? (Work, Family & others)

_____
_____
_____
_____
_____
_____

## Steps towards your goals

_____
_____
_____
_____
_____
_____
_____

**Date:**

### Triggers / Environment

_____
_____
_____
_____
_____
_____
_____

### Symptoms

_____
_____
_____
_____
_____
_____

### Medication / Support System

_____
_____
_____
_____
_____
_____
_____

**Stay Active**                                    **Date:**

## Activity / Workout / Creativity / Hobbies

_____
_____
_____
_____
_____
_____
_____
_____

## What are your goals ? (Work, Family & others)

_____
_____
_____
_____
_____
_____

## Steps towards your goals

_____
_____
_____
_____
_____
_____
_____

**Date:**

Triggers / Environment
_____
_____
_____
_____
_____
_____
_____
_____

Symptoms
_____
_____
_____
_____
_____
_____
_____
_____

Medication / Support System
_____
_____
_____
_____
_____
_____
_____
_____

**Stay Active**  **Date:**

Activity / Workout / Creativity / Hobbies
___

What are your goals ? (Work, Family & others)
___

Steps towards your goals
___

**Date:**

## Triggers / Environment

## Symptoms

## Medication / Support System

**Stay Active**  Date:

Activity / Workout / Creativity / Hobbies
_____

_____
_____
_____
_____
_____
_____
_____

What are your goals ? (Work, Family & others)
_____

_____
_____
_____
_____
_____
_____
_____

Steps towards your goals
_____

_____
_____
_____
_____
_____
_____
_____

**Date:**

## Triggers / Environment

_____
_____
_____
_____
_____
_____
_____

## Symptoms

_____
_____
_____
_____
_____
_____
_____

## Medication / Support System

_____
_____
_____
_____
_____
_____
_____

# Stay Active

**Date:**

## Activity / Workout / Creativity / Hobbies

_____
_____
_____
_____
_____
_____
_____
_____

## What are your goals ? (Work, Family & others)

_____
_____
_____
_____
_____
_____
_____

## Steps towards your goals

_____
_____
_____
_____
_____
_____
_____

**Date:**

### Triggers / Environment

_____
_____
_____
_____
_____
_____
_____

### Symptoms

_____
_____
_____
_____
_____
_____
_____

### Medication / Support System

_____
_____
_____
_____
_____
_____
_____

# Stay Active

**Date:**

## Activity / Workout / Creativity / Hobbies

_____
_____
_____
_____
_____
_____
_____

## What are your goals ? (Work, Family & others)

_____
_____
_____
_____
_____
_____
_____

## Steps towards your goals

_____
_____
_____
_____
_____
_____
_____

**Date:**

## Triggers / Environment

## Symptoms

## Medication / Support System

**Stay Active**                              **Date:**

Activity / Workout / Creativity / Hobbies
_____

_____
_____
_____
_____
_____
_____

What are your goals ? (Work, Family & others)
_____

_____
_____
_____
_____
_____
_____

Steps towards your goals
_____

_____
_____
_____
_____
_____
_____

**Date:**

### Triggers / Environment

_____
_____
_____
_____
_____
_____
_____

### Symptoms

_____
_____
_____
_____
_____
_____
_____

### Medication / Support System

_____
_____
_____
_____
_____
_____
_____

**Stay Active**　　　　　　　　　　**Date:**

Activity / Workout / Creativity / Hobbies
_____

_____
_____
_____
_____
_____
_____
_____

What are your goals ? (Work, Family & others)
_____

_____
_____
_____
_____
_____
_____

Steps towards your goals
_____

_____
_____
_____
_____
_____
_____
_____

**Date:**

## Triggers / Environment

## Symptoms

## Medication / Support System

**Stay Active**                    **Date:**

Activity / Workout / Creativity / Hobbies
_____
_____
_____
_____
_____
_____
_____

What are your goals ? (Work, Family & others)
_____
_____
_____
_____
_____
_____
_____

Steps towards your goals
_____
_____
_____
_____
_____
_____
_____

**Date:**

Triggers / Environment

Symptoms

Medication / Support System

# Stay Active                    Date:

## Activity / Workout / Creativity / Hobbies

_____
_____
_____
_____
_____
_____
_____

## What are your goals ? (Work, Family & others)

_____
_____
_____
_____
_____
_____
_____

## Steps towards your goals

_____
_____
_____
_____
_____
_____
_____

**Date:**

## Triggers / Environment

## Symptoms

## Medication / Support System

**Stay Active**                                    **Date:**

Activity / Workout / Creativity / Hobbies
_____

_____
_____
_____
_____
_____
_____
_____

What are your goals ? (Work, Family & others)
_____

_____
_____
_____
_____
_____
_____

Steps towards your goals
_____

_____
_____
_____
_____
_____
_____
_____

**Date:**

Triggers / Environment
_____
_____
_____
_____
_____
_____
_____
_____

Symptoms
_____
_____
_____
_____
_____
_____
_____
_____

Medication / Support System
_____
_____
_____
_____
_____
_____
_____
_____
_____

**Stay Active**                    **Date:**

Activity / Workout / Creativity / Hobbies
_____
_____
_____
_____
_____
_____
_____
_____

What are your goals ? (Work, Family & others)
_____
_____
_____
_____
_____
_____
_____

Steps towards your goals
_____
_____
_____
_____
_____
_____
_____

**Date:**

### Triggers / Environment

### Symptoms

### Medication / Support System

# Stay Active

**Date:**

Activity / Workout / Creativity / Hobbies

___

What are your goals? (Work, Family & others)

___

Steps towards your goals

___

**Date:**

Triggers / Environment

Symptoms

Medication / Support System

# Stay Active

**Date:**

## Activity / Workout / Creativity / Hobbies

_____
_____
_____
_____
_____
_____
_____
_____

## What are your goals ? (Work, Family & others)

_____
_____
_____
_____
_____
_____
_____

## Steps towards your goals

_____
_____
_____
_____
_____
_____
_____

**Date:**

Triggers / Environment
_____
_____
_____
_____
_____
_____
_____
_____

Symptoms
_____
_____
_____
_____
_____
_____
_____
_____

Medication / Support System
_____
_____
_____
_____
_____
_____
_____
_____

**Stay Active**                         **Date:**

Activity / Workout / Creativity / Hobbies
_____
_____
_____
_____
_____
_____
_____
_____

What are your goals ? (Work, Family & others)
_____
_____
_____
_____
_____
_____
_____

Steps towards your goals
_____
_____
_____
_____
_____
_____
_____

**Date:**

Triggers / Environment

Symptoms

Medication / Support System

# Stay Active                    Date:

## Activity / Workout / Creativity / Hobbies

_____
_____
_____
_____
_____
_____
_____

## What are your goals ? (Work, Family & others)

_____
_____
_____
_____
_____
_____
_____

## Steps towards your goals

_____
_____
_____
_____
_____
_____
_____

**Date:**

## Triggers / Environment

## Symptoms

## Medication / Support System

**Stay Active**                    **Date:**

Activity / Workout / Creativity / Hobbies
_____
_____
_____
_____
_____
_____
_____
_____

What are your goals ? (Work, Family & others)
_____
_____
_____
_____
_____
_____
_____
_____

Steps towards your goals
_____
_____
_____
_____
_____
_____
_____
_____

**Date:**

Triggers / Environment
_____
_____
_____
_____
_____
_____
_____

Symptoms
_____
_____
_____
_____
_____
_____
_____

Medication / Support System
_____
_____
_____
_____
_____
_____
_____

**Stay Active**                                **Date:**

Activity / Workout / Creativity / Hobbies
_____

_____
_____
_____
_____
_____
_____
_____

What are your goals ? (Work, Family & others)
_____

_____
_____
_____
_____
_____
_____

Steps towards your goals
_____

_____
_____
_____
_____
_____
_____
_____

**Date:**

## Triggers / Environment

_____
_____
_____
_____
_____
_____
_____

## Symptoms

_____
_____
_____
_____
_____
_____
_____

## Medication / Support System

_____
_____
_____
_____
_____
_____
_____

**Stay Active**  **Date:**

Activity / Workout / Creativity / Hobbies
_____
_____
_____
_____
_____
_____
_____

What are your goals ? (Work, Family & others)
_____
_____
_____
_____
_____
_____
_____

Steps towards your goals
_____
_____
_____
_____
_____
_____
_____

**Date:**

Triggers / Environment

Symptoms

Medication / Support System

**Stay Active**                                **Date:**

Activity / Workout / Creativity / Hobbies
_____

_____
_____
_____
_____
_____
_____
_____

What are your goals ? (Work, Family & others)
_____

_____
_____
_____
_____
_____
_____

Steps towards your goals
_____

_____
_____
_____
_____
_____
_____
_____

**Date:**

### Triggers / Environment

_____
_____
_____
_____
_____
_____
_____

### Symptoms

_____
_____
_____
_____
_____
_____
_____

### Medication / Support System

_____
_____
_____
_____
_____
_____
_____

**Stay Active**  **Date:**

Activity / Workout / Creativity / Hobbies
___
___
___
___
___
___
___
___

What are your goals ? (Work, Family & others)
___
___
___
___
___
___
___
___

Steps towards your goals
___
___
___
___
___
___
___
___

**Date:**

Triggers / Environment

Symptoms

Medication / Support System

**Stay Active**                              **Date:**

Activity / Workout / Creativity / Hobbies
_____

_____
_____
_____
_____
_____
_____
_____

What are your goals ? (Work, Family & others)
_____

_____
_____
_____
_____
_____
_____
_____

Steps towards your goals
_____

_____
_____
_____
_____
_____
_____
_____

**Date:**

### Triggers / Environment

---
---
---
---
---
---
---

### Symptoms

---
---
---
---
---
---
---

### Medication / Support System

---
---
---
---
---
---
---

**Stay Active**                    **Date:**

Activity / Workout / Creativity / Hobbies

_____

_____

_____

_____

_____

_____

_____

What are your goals ? (Work, Family & others)

_____

_____

_____

_____

_____

_____

_____

Steps towards your goals

_____

_____

_____

_____

_____

_____

_____

**Date:**

Triggers / Environment
_____
_____
_____
_____
_____
_____
_____
_____

Symptoms
_____
_____
_____
_____
_____
_____
_____
_____

Medication / Support System
_____
_____
_____
_____
_____
_____
_____
_____

**Stay Active**                              **Date:**

Activity / Workout / Creativity / Hobbies
_____
_____
_____
_____
_____
_____
_____
_____

What are your goals ? (Work, Family & others)
_____
_____
_____
_____
_____
_____
_____

Steps towards your goals
_____
_____
_____
_____
_____
_____
_____
_____

**Date:**

### Triggers / Environment

_____
_____
_____
_____
_____
_____
_____

### Symptoms

_____
_____
_____
_____
_____
_____
_____

### Medication / Support System

_____
_____
_____
_____
_____
_____
_____

# Stay Active

**Date:**

## Activity / Workout / Creativity / Hobbies

___

## What are your goals ? (Work, Family & others)

___

## Steps towards your goals

___

**Date:**

Triggers / Environment
___

Symptoms
___

Medication / Support System
___

**Stay Active**                               **Date:**

Activity / Workout / Creativity / Hobbies
_____

_____
_____
_____
_____
_____
_____
_____

What are your goals ? (Work, Family & others)
_____

_____
_____
_____
_____
_____
_____

Steps towards your goals
_____

_____
_____
_____
_____
_____
_____
_____

**Date:**

Triggers / Environment
_____
_____
_____
_____
_____
_____
_____
_____

Symptoms
_____
_____
_____
_____
_____
_____
_____
_____

Medication / Support System
_____
_____
_____
_____
_____
_____
_____
_____

**Stay Active**                    **Date:**

Activity / Workout / Creativity / Hobbies

What are your goals ? (Work, Family & others)

Steps towards your goals

**Date:**

### Triggers / Environment

---
---
---
---
---
---
---
---

### Symptoms

---
---
---
---
---
---
---
---

### Medication / Support System

---
---
---
---
---
---
---
---

**Stay Active**  **Date:**

Activity / Workout / Creativity / Hobbies
_____
_____
_____
_____
_____
_____
_____
_____

What are your goals ? (Work, Family & others)
_____
_____
_____
_____
_____
_____
_____
_____

Steps towards your goals
_____
_____
_____
_____
_____
_____
_____
_____

**Date:**

Triggers / Environment
___

Symptoms
___

Medication / Support System
___

**Stay Active**                                   **Date:**

Activity / Workout / Creativity / Hobbies
_____

_____
_____
_____
_____
_____
_____
_____

What are your goals ? (Work, Family & others)
_____

_____
_____
_____
_____
_____
_____

Steps towards your goals
_____

_____
_____
_____
_____
_____
_____

**Date:**

### Triggers / Environment

_____
_____
_____
_____
_____
_____
_____

### Symptoms

_____
_____
_____
_____
_____
_____
_____

### Medication / Support System

_____
_____
_____
_____
_____
_____
_____

**Stay Active**  **Date:**

Activity / Workout / Creativity / Hobbies
_____
_____
_____
_____
_____
_____
_____
_____

What are your goals ? (Work, Family & others)
_____
_____
_____
_____
_____
_____
_____

Steps towards your goals
_____
_____
_____
_____
_____
_____
_____
_____

**Date:**

## Triggers / Environment

## Symptoms

## Medication / Support System

# Stay Active

**Date:**

## Activity / Workout / Creativity / Hobbies

_____
_____
_____
_____
_____
_____
_____

## What are your goals ? (Work, Family & others)

_____
_____
_____
_____
_____
_____
_____

## Steps towards your goals

_____
_____
_____
_____
_____
_____
_____

**Date:**

Triggers / Environment
_____
_____
_____
_____
_____
_____
_____

Symptoms
_____
_____
_____
_____
_____
_____
_____

Medication / Support System
_____
_____
_____
_____
_____
_____
_____

**Stay Active**            **Date:**

Activity / Workout / Creativity / Hobbies

What are your goals ? (Work, Family & others)

Steps towards your goals

**Date:**

Triggers / Environment

Symptoms

Medication / Support System

**Stay Active**　　　　　　　　　　**Date:**

Activity / Workout / Creativity / Hobbies
___

What are your goals ? (Work, Family & others)
___

Steps towards your goals
___

**Date:**

## Triggers / Environment

## Symptoms

## Medication / Support System

# Stay Active

**Date:**

## Activity / Workout / Creativity / Hobbies

_____
_____
_____
_____
_____
_____
_____

## What are your goals ? (Work, Family & others)

_____
_____
_____
_____
_____
_____
_____

## Steps towards your goals

_____
_____
_____
_____
_____
_____
_____

**Date:**

Triggers / Environment

Symptoms

Medication / Support System

# Stay Active

**Date:**

## Activity / Workout / Creativity / Hobbies

_____
_____
_____
_____
_____
_____
_____

## What are your goals ? (Work, Family & others)

_____
_____
_____
_____
_____
_____
_____

## Steps towards your goals

_____
_____
_____
_____
_____
_____
_____

**Date:**

### Triggers / Environment

_____
_____
_____
_____
_____
_____
_____

### Symptoms

_____
_____
_____
_____
_____
_____

### Medication / Support System

_____
_____
_____
_____
_____
_____
_____

**Stay Active**                    **Date:**

Activity / Workout / Creativity / Hobbies

_____
_____
_____
_____
_____
_____
_____

What are your goals ? (Work, Family & others)

_____
_____
_____
_____
_____
_____
_____

Steps towards your goals

_____
_____
_____
_____
_____
_____
_____

**Date:**

## Triggers / Environment

## Symptoms

## Medication / Support System

# Stay Active

**Date:**

## Activity / Workout / Creativity / Hobbies

---

## What are your goals ? (Work, Family & others)

---

## Steps towards your goals

**Date:**

### Triggers / Environment

_____
_____
_____
_____
_____
_____
_____

### Symptoms

_____
_____
_____
_____
_____
_____
_____

### Medication / Support System

_____
_____
_____
_____
_____
_____
_____

**Stay Active**              **Date:**

Activity / Workout / Creativity / Hobbies

_____
_____
_____
_____
_____
_____
_____

What are your goals ? (Work, Family & others)

_____
_____
_____
_____
_____
_____

Steps towards your goals

_____
_____
_____
_____
_____
_____
_____

**Date:**

Triggers / Environment
_____
_____
_____
_____
_____
_____
_____

Symptoms
_____
_____
_____
_____
_____
_____
_____

Medication / Support System
_____
_____
_____
_____
_____
_____
_____
_____

**Stay Active**　　　　　　　　　　**Date:**

Activity / Workout / Creativity / Hobbies
_____
_____
_____
_____
_____
_____
_____
_____

What are your goals ? (Work, Family & others)
_____
_____
_____
_____
_____
_____
_____
_____

Steps towards your goals
_____
_____
_____
_____
_____
_____
_____
_____

**Date:**

## Triggers / Environment

_____
_____
_____
_____
_____
_____
_____
_____

## Symptoms

_____
_____
_____
_____
_____
_____
_____
_____

## Medication / Support System

_____
_____
_____
_____
_____
_____
_____
_____

# Stay Active

**Date:**

## Activity / Workout / Creativity / Hobbies

___

___

___

___

___

___

___

## What are your goals ? (Work, Family & others)

___

___

___

___

___

___

___

## Steps towards your goals

___

___

___

___

___

___

___

___

**Date:**

Triggers / Environment
_____
_____
_____
_____
_____
_____
_____

Symptoms
_____
_____
_____
_____
_____
_____
_____

Medication / Support System
_____
_____
_____
_____
_____
_____
_____

**Stay Active**  **Date:**

Activity / Workout / Creativity / Hobbies
_____
_____
_____
_____
_____
_____
_____
_____

What are your goals ? (Work, Family & others)
_____
_____
_____
_____
_____
_____
_____

Steps towards your goals
_____
_____
_____
_____
_____
_____
_____
_____

**Date:**

## Triggers / Environment

_____
_____
_____
_____
_____
_____
_____
_____

## Symptoms

_____
_____
_____
_____
_____
_____
_____
_____

## Medication / Support System

_____
_____
_____
_____
_____
_____
_____
_____

**Stay Active**                        **Date:**

Activity / Workout / Creativity / Hobbies

___

___

___

___

___

___

___

What are your goals ? (Work, Family & others)

___

___

___

___

___

___

___

Steps towards your goals

___

___

___

___

___

___

___

**Date:**

Triggers / Environment

Symptoms

Medication / Support System

**Stay Active**　　　　　　　　　　**Date:**

Activity / Workout / Creativity / Hobbies

---
---
---
---
---
---
---

What are your goals ? (Work, Family & others)

---
---
---
---
---
---
---

Steps towards your goals

---
---
---
---
---
---
---

**Date:**

## Triggers / Environment

## Symptoms

## Medication / Support System

**Stay Active**  **Date:**

Activity / Workout / Creativity / Hobbies

---
---
---
---
---
---
---

What are your goals ? (Work, Family & others)

---
---
---
---
---
---
---

Steps towards your goals

---
---
---
---
---
---
---

**Date:**

## Triggers / Environment

_____
_____
_____
_____
_____
_____
_____

## Symptoms

_____
_____
_____
_____
_____
_____

## Medication / Support System

_____
_____
_____
_____
_____
_____
_____
_____

**Stay Active**  **Date:**

Activity / Workout / Creativity / Hobbies

What are your goals ? (Work, Family & others)

Steps towards your goals

**Date:**

### Triggers / Environment

### Symptoms

### Medication / Support System

www.ingramcontent.com/pod-product-compliance
Lightning Source LLC
Chambersburg PA
CBHW070433220526
45466CB00004B/1657